30-Day Ketogenic Diet Plan

Lose weight in the most effective way

Matthew Knoll

© 2016

TABLE OF CONTENTS

INTRODUCTION

Beginning with Keto diet is not easy; it requires tremendous determination and a lot of effort. However, as they say, nothing can beat the human determination. If you decide to make your body lean with Ketogenic diet and follow it with complete dedication, nothing can stop you. The best part about Ketogenic diet is that you do not have to count your calories while indulging in all the meats and fats.

You can eat as much as you want and your body will automatically adapt to use fats as energy in place of carbohydrates. You are free from all kinds of worries. Just concentrate your mind on adapting to your new diet since you will definitely crave for sugar and carbohydrates in the initial few weeks.

Ketogenic diet has several benefits and the most important of them being losing weight quickly. It is especially beneficial for those who aim to lose significant weight and those who are into weight training.

This book gives you a diet plan for complete 30 days so that you do not have to get up every morning and think *what to eat!* This should be the last thing to worry on your agenda. This book relieves you from a major tension and lets you concentrate on other important things. In 30 days, you can easily adapt to this diet. By the end of a month, you can yourself invent new cuisines and go ahead.

Day 1

Breakfast- Poppy seed Lemon Muffins

Yields	:	12 cupcakes
Preparation time	:	20 minutes
Total time	:	30-40 minutes

Ingredients:

Flaxseed meal	¼ cup
Almond flour	¾ cup
Poppy seeds	2 tablespoons
Erythitol	1/3 cup
Heavy cream	¼ cup
Salted butter	¼ cup
Eggs	3 large
Vanilla extract	1 teaspoon
Lemon zest	2 lemons
Lemon juice	3 tablespoons
Stevia	25 drops

Directions:

Take a bowl and combine flaxseed meal, almond flour, poppy seeds, and erythitol. Add heavy cream, and eggs to make a smooth mixture. Add vanilla, baking powder, lemon zest, lemon juice, and stevia. Divide the mixture into 12 molds of cupcakes and bake them in a preheated oven at a temperature of 350F. Bake for 20 minutes until the cupcakes are browned. Take out the molds and let cool. Slice before serving.

Lunch- Mexican dip

Yields	:	2
Preparation time	:	20 minutes
Total time	:	40 minutes

Ingredients for guac:

Pitted, peeled, ripe avocados	2
Lime juice	1 tablespoon
Fresh cilantro	¼ cup
Chopped White onion	¼ cup
Cherry tomatoes	6
Minced garlic	1 teaspoon

| Sea salt | ½ teaspoon |

Ingredients for beef:

Ground beef	2 pounds
Water	½ cup
Taco seasoning	¼ cup
Organic sour cream	2 cups
Shredded lettuce	2 cups
Cheddar cheese	2 cups
Cayenne pepper	as per taste

Directions:

Take a bowl to combine avocado, cilantro, limejuice, onion, garlic, tomato, and salt. Refrigerate while you prepare beef. Cook ground beef in a skillet over medium flame to crumble it. Add water, stir it, and then add taco seasoning. Simmer the heat and cook for ten minutes. Take out the beef into bowls and top them with sour cream. Add guacamole from the refrigerator, lettuce, cheddar cheese, and drizzle cayenne pepper. Serve.

Dinner – Cheeseburger Bacon Waffles

Yields	:	3-4
Preparation time	:	20
Total time	:	40 min

Ingredients (for waffles):

Cheddar cheese	1.5 ounce
Eggs	2 large
Cauliflower crumbles	cauliflower crumbles
Garlic powder	¼ teaspoon
Onion powder	¼ teaspoon
Almond flour	4 tablespoons
Parmesan cheese	3 tablespoons
Pepper	as per taste
Salt	as per taste

Ingredients (for topping):

Ground beef	4 ounce
Chopped bacon	4 slices
Barbeque sauce	4 tablespoons
Cheddar cheese	1.5 ounces

| Pepper | as per taste |
| Salt | as per taste |

Directions:

For making waffles, collect cheddar cheese, eggs, cauliflower crumbles, garlic powder, onion powder, almond flour, parmesan cheese, pepper, and salt. For topping, collect ground beef, chopped bacon, barbeque sauce, cheddar cheese, pepper, and salt. Combine shredded cheddar cheese, eggs, parmesan cheese, spices, and almond flour, and keep it aside as waffle mixture. Slice thin pieces of bacon over high- medium heat. After the bacon is cooked partially, add beef and let cook. Take out the excessive fat from the frying pan to the waffle mixture. Blend the waffle mixture using immersion blender. Put the waffle mixture into the waffle iron to make it crisp. When the steam stops coming from the waffle iron, take it out. Add barbeque sauce into the beef and bacon mixture. Add the beef mixture to the waffles, top it with cheddar cheese, broil for a couple of minutes to melt the cheese. Serve.

Day 2

Breakfast- Pizza Frittata

Yields	:	2-3
Preparation time	:	20 min
Total time	:	45-50 min

Ingredients:

Frozen spinach	90 ounce
Olive oil	4 tablespoon
Nutmeg	¼ teaspoon
Eggs	12 large
Parmesan cheese	½ cup
Ricotta cheese	½ cup
Mozzarella cheese	5 ounce
Pepperoni	1 ounce
Minced garlic	1 teaspoon
Salt	as per taste
Pepper	as per taste

Directions:

Thaw frozen spinach in microwave for 4 minutes and drain out water. Combine olive oil, spices, and eggs. Add parmesan, ricotta, and spinach (broken into pieces). Put this mixture into an iron skillet, and add mozzarella cheese and pepperoni afterwards in the skillet over the mixture. Bake the mixture for 30 minutes in a preheated oven at 375F. Take out and serve.

Lunch- Cheese Crust Pizza

Yields	:	2-3
Preparation time	:	20 min
Total time	:	30 min

Ingredients:

Ground beef	1 pound
Beef hot dog	2 organic
4-cheese blend	1.5 cups
Shredded cheddar	1.5 cups
Paprika	¼ tablespoon
Sea salt	¼ teaspoon
Ground black pepper	¼ teaspoon

Old bay	¼ teaspoon
Garlic powder	¼ teaspoon
Onion powder	¼ teaspoon
Thousand island dressing	1 tablespoon
Chopped romaine	1 cup
Yellow onions	2 tablespoons
Chopped dill pickle	2 tablespoon
Shredded American cheese	½ cup
Low sugar ketchup	as per taste
Mustard	as per taste

Directions:

Layer cheese blend in a non-stick frying pan greased with virgin olive oil. Add another layer of shredded cheddar. Cook for 5 minutes, lift its edges with a spatula, and take it out on an even surface. Let cool. Add Thousand Island dressing onto the crust. Cook hamburger in the skillet to brown it. Add sea salt, paprika, ground black pepper, garlic powder, old bay seasoning, a little water, and onion powder. Combine well and simmer the heat. Chop the hot dogs and add them to the mixture. Cook for 5 minutes. Put chopped lettuce on the pizza crust. Chop pickles, onions and shred American cheese. Add the hamburger mixture onto lettuce, add chopped pickles mixture, drizzle mustard and ketchup and sprinkle American cheese. Serve.

Dinner- Chicken Tikka

Yields	:	3-4
Preparation time	:	20 min
Total time	:	6 hours 20 min

Ingredients:

Chicken thighs with bones	1.5 pounds
Boneless chicken thighs	1 pound
Olive oil	2 tablespoon
Onion powder	2 teaspoons
Minced garlic	3 cloves
Grated ginger root	1 inch
Tomato paste	3 tablespoon
Indian spice mixture	5 teaspoons
Smoked paprika	2 teaspoons
Kosher salt	4 teaspoons
Diced tomatoes	10 ounces
Coconut milk	1 cup

| Chopped cilantro | for topping |
| Guar gum | 1 teaspoon |

Directions:

Collect chicken thighs with bones, boneless chicken thighs, olive oil, onion powder, minced garlic, grated ginger root, tomato paste, Indian spice mixture, smoked paprika, kosher salt, diced tomatoes, coconut milk, chopped cilantro, and guar gum. Remove bones from the chicken thighs, chop them into small pieces, and keep the skin. Put it into slow cooker along with grated ginger and dry spices. Add tomatoes, tomato paste, and coconut milk, and set the slow cooker on low. Mix the ingredients and cook for 6 hours. After the chicken is cooked, add residual coconut milk, guar gum, heavy cream, and stir. Serve it with cauliflower rice.

Day 3

Breakfast- Low Carb Casserole

Yields   :   2-3
Preparation time :   10 min
Total time   :   65 min

Ingredients:

Breakfast sausage	2
Almond flour	2 cups
Flaxseed meal	1.5 cups
Eggs	2
Cheese	1.5 cups
Maple syrup	2 tablespoons
Butter	2 tablespoons
Onion powder	1 teaspoon
Garlic powder	¼ teaspoon
Sage	as per taste

Directions:

Heat a pan, add breakfast sausage to it, and break it into pieces. Collect almond flour, flaxseed meal, eggs, cheese, maple syrup, butter, onion powder, garlic powder, and sage. Take a bowl and mix dry ingredients. Now, combine wet ingredients into it. After the sausage gains brown color, add the mixture to it, and stir well. In a casserole dish lined with parchment paper, pour this mixture. Bake it in a preheated oven at 350F for 50-55 minutes. Take out, let cool, remove from the dish, and serve.

Lunch- Beef Burger

Yields	:	2- 3
Preparation time	:	5 min
Total time	:	35 min

Ingredients:

Ground beef (80%)	1 pound
Ground brisket	1 pound
Plain mayo	2 tablespoons

Minced Garlic	1 tablespoon
Butter	½ stick, cut into eight slices
Olive oil	1 tablespoon
Yellow Onion	1 large
Ghee	1 tablespoon
Your favorite seasonings	

Directions:

Combine brisket and beef. Add everything seasoning, plain mayo, and garlic. Combine well. Make patties of this mixture. Make small pockets in patties and pack them with butter, and seal them back. Heat olive oil in cast iron frying pan, sauté onions, add some water and mix. Corner the onions in the pan. Add patties to the frying pan and cook them on low- medium heat for 20 minutes. Flatten the burgers and brown them on each side. Add ghee if required. Keep shuffling the onions and take them out when they are ready. Take out the burgers and onions in a plate and top them with cheese. Serve.

Dinner- Chili Soup

Yields	:	2-3
Preparation time	:	5 min
Total time	:	30 min

Ingredients:

Chicken thighs	16 ounces
Chicken broth	2 cups
Pepper	as per taste
Salt	as per taste
Coriander seeds	1 teaspoon
Sliced chili peppers	2
Water	2 cups
Ground cumin	½ teaspoon
Turmeric	1 teaspoon
Butter	2 tablespoons
Tomato paste	4 tablespoons
Lemon juice	half lime
Avocado	1 medium
Chopped Cilantro	4 tablespoons
Quesco fresco	2 ounces

Directions:

Put the chicken thighs in a greased frying pan. Season it with pepper and salt, and let it cook. Put coriander seeds and sliced chili peppers to release more flavors. Add water and broth and let it simmer. Add ground cumin, turmeric, pepper, and salt, and let cook. Add butter and tomato paste, and stir. Simmer for 5-10 minutes. Add lemon juice. Put the chicken thighs at the base of bowl and pour soup from the top. Garnish with avocado, cilantro, and quesco fresco.

Day 4

Breakfast- Keto Brownie Muffins

Yields	:	2- 3
Preparation time	:	5- 10 min
Total time	:	30 min

Ingredients:

Flaxseed meal	1 cup
Cocoa powder	¼ cup
Cinnamon powder	1 tablespoon
Baking powder	½ tablespoon
Egg	1 large
Salt	½ teaspoons
Coconut oil	2 tablespoon
Caramel syrup	¼ cup
Pumpkin purees	½ cup
Vanilla extract	1 teaspoon
Apple cider vinegar	1 teaspoon
Slivered almonds	¼ cup

Muffin liners

Paper liners

Directions:

You need flaxseed meal, cocoa powder, cinnamon powder, baking powder, egg, salt, coconut oil, caramel syrup, pumpkin puree, vanilla extract, apple cider vinegar, and slivered almonds. Take a bowl and combine all the ingredients. Take muffin liners and spoon each of them with 6 paper liners. Drop slivered almonds on the top and press lightly. Bake it in a preheated oven at 350F for 15 minutes until the muffins rise.

Lunch- Banana Peppers Stuffed with Sausage

Yields	:	2- 3
Preparation time	:	15 min
Total time	:	30- 40 min

Ingredients:

Banana peppers	4
Olive oil	2 tablespoons

Sweet Sausages	1 pound
Ghee	1 tablespoon
Herbs	½ teaspoon
Onions	3 tablespoons
Mozzarella cheese	as per requirement
Marinara sauce	2 tablespoons

Directions:

Rub banana peppers with olive oil and bake them in a preheated oven at 350F or 20 minutes. Cook sausages in a skillet over medium heat. Add ghee, herbs, and onions, and cook over low heat for 5 minutes. Take out the banana peppers and turn on the broiler at 500. Stuff the banana peppers with mixture of sausage and top them using mozzarella cheese. Now, place the peppers on a cookie sheet with a thin marinara layer. Bake for 5-10 minutes to make mozzarella bubble. Take out and serve.

Dinner- Pumpkin Carbonara

| Yields | : | 2- 3 |
| Preparation time | : | 10 min |

Total time   :   25 min

Ingredients:

Shirataki noodles	1 package
Chopped pancetta	5 ounce
Butter	2 tablespoon
Dried Sage	½ teaspoon
Pumpkins puree	3 tablespoon
Heavy cream	¼ cup
Parmesan cheese	1/3 cup
Egg yolks	2 large

Directions:

Drain Shirataki noodles in hot water stream for 3 minutes. Dry them using paper towels. Put chopped pancetta into a hot pan. Take a pan and melt butter in it. After it browns, add sage and mix. Add pumpkin puree to cook. When the pancetta browns, take it out of the pan and keep its fat aside. Put heavy cream in the sauce and mix well. Put the pancetta's fat in the sauce, stir well and simmer the heat. Raise the heat of pancetta to high, add shirataki noodles, and dry fry the noodles for 5 minutes. When the steam starts coming out from the pan, turn off the heat. Put parmesan cheese into pumpkin sauce, stir well, and simmer the heat. Keep stirring the sauce. When the sauce thickens, add noodles to the sauce. Toss the noodles, add 2 egg yolks to the pan, and mix well. Serve with parmesan cheese.

Day 5

Breakfast- Keto Tacos

Yields	:	2- 3
Preparation time	:	15 min
Total time	:	35 min

Ingredients:

Bacon	3 strips
Mozzarella cheese	1 cup
Eggs	6 large
Butter	2 tablespoon
Pepper	as per taste
Salt	as per taste
Avocado	½ small
Cheddar cheese	1 ounce
Cilantro	for topping

Directions:

Bake some pieces of bacon on the baking sheet lined with aluminum foil for 15-20 minutes at a temperature of 375F. As the bacon cooks, heat mozzarella on average heat for 2-3 minutes to make taco shells. When the cheese browns on its edges, lift it, drape it on top of the handle of a horizontally hanging wooden ladle. Cook some eggs in butter, season with pepper and salt, and spoon them along with bacon and avocado in the taco shells. Dust cheddar cheese, cilantro, and sauce on top of the tacos.

Lunch- Broccoli Cheese Pizza

Yields	:	2- 3
Preparation time	:	15 min
Total time	:	25 min

Ingredients:

Garlic Olive oil	1 tablespoon
Pizza cheese	1 cup
Mozzarella cheese	1 cup
Ghee	2 tablespoon

Mascarpone cheese	¼ cup
Minced Garlic	1 teaspoon
Heavy cream	1 tablespoon
Salt	as per taste
Pepper	as per taste
Chopped steamed Broccoli	1/3 cup
Asiago cheese	as per taste
Pepper lemon seasoning	as per taste

Directions:

Heat olive oil in a non-stick frying pan. Put pizza cheese blend and make a pizza crust out of it. Add a layer of mozzarella cheese and cook for 5 minutes to make it crisp. Use a wooden spatula to take off the edges from the pan and take it out on a even surface. Let cool. Add ghee, mascarpone cheese, garlic, heavy cream, salt, and lemon pepper to the heated pan. Cook for 5 minutes to let the mixture bubble. Drizzle half of this mixture onto the crust. Put some steamed chopped broccoli to the remaining mixture. Cook for a minute and add it to the pizza. Now, sprinkle asiago cheese, pepper lemon seasoning on the top, and serve.

Dinner- Crusted Salmon with Walnuts

Yields	:	2- 3
Preparation time	:	15-20 min
Total time	:	30 min

Ingredients:

Walnuts	½ cup
Spices of your choice	
Maple syrup	1 tablespoon
Dill	¼ teaspoon
Dijon mustard	1 tablespoon
Dried salmon fillets	2/3 ounce

Directions:

Pulse half a cup walnuts in food processor. Add your favorite spices and maple syrup, and stir. Add mustard sauce and pulse the mixture to make a paste. Heat oil in a skillet on high and place dried salmon fillets in the pan and let cook for 3 minutes. Put walnut mixture over the salmon. After the salmon has seared, move it to a preheated oven at 350F and bake for 8 minutes. Serve with spinach and sprinkle smoked paprika.

DAY 6

Breakfast- Keto Tacos

Yields	:	2- 3
Preparation time	:	25 min
Total time	:	35 min

Ingredients:

Bacon	3 strips
Mozzarella cheese	1 cup
Eggs	6 large
Butter	2 tablespoons
Pepper	as per taste
Salt	as per taste
Avocado	½ small
Cheddar cheese	1 ounce
Cilantro	for topping

Directions:

Bake some pieces of bacon on the baking sheet lined with aluminum foil for 15-20 minutes at a temperature of 375F. As the bacon cooks, heat mozzarella on average heat for 2-3 minutes to make taco shells. When the cheese browns on its edges, lift it, drape it on top of the handle of a horizontally hanging wooden ladle. Cook some eggs in butter, season with pepper and salt, and spoon them along with bacon and avocado in the taco shells. Dust cheddar cheese, cilantro, and sauce on top of the tacos.

Lunch- Zuchhini Noodles Salad

Yields	:	2
Preparation time	:	5 min
Total time	:	10 min

Ingredients:

Zucchini noodles	2 cups
Fresh spinach	1 cup
Bleu cheese, Crumbled	1/3 cup
Crumbled bacon	½ cup
Bleu cheese dressing	1/3 cup
Cracked pepper	as per taste
Broccoli	as per taste

Directions:

Collect zucchini noodles, fresh spinach, cheese dressing, crumbled cheese, crumbled bacon, and cracked pepper. Toss these ingredients, add broccoli, and enjoy.

Dinner- Braised Oxtails

Yields	:	2- 3
Preparation time	:	30 min
Total time	:	7 hours 30 min

Ingredients:

Beef broth	2 cup
Soy sauce	2 tablespoon
Tomato paste	3 tablespoon
Butter	1/3 cup
Fish sauce	1 tablespoon
Oxtails	2 pounds
Onion powder	1 tablespoon
Ground ginger	½ teaspoon

Pepper	as per taste
Salt	as per taste
Dried thyme	1 teaspoon
Guar gum	½ teaspoon
Cauliflower mashed potatoes	

Directions:

Heat beef broth over high, add soy sauce, tomato paste, butter, fish sauce to the pan, and mix well. Take it out into slow cooker and let the mixture heat up. Place oxtails over the mixture and season them with minced garlic, onion powder, ground ginger, pepper, salt, and dried thyme. Set the slow cooker on low and let cook for 7 hours. Take out the oxtails on paper towels in order to drain. Blend the juices of slow cooker using immersion blender. Add a little guar gum and serve with some cauliflower mashed potatoes and gravy.

Day 7

Breakfast- Pizza Waffles

Yields	:	2- 3
Preparation time	:	10 min
Total time	:	15-25 min

Ingredients:

Eggs	4 large
Parmesan cheese	4 tablespoon
Almond flour	3 tablespoon
Husk powder	1 tablespoon
Butter	1 tablespoon
Baking powder	1 teaspoon
Italian seasoning	1 teaspoon
Pepper	as per taste
Salt	as per taste
Tomato sauce	½ cup
Cheddar cheese	3 ounces
Pepperoni	14 slices

Directions:

Collect eggs, parmesan cheese, almond flour, husk powder, butter, baking powder, Italian seasoning, pepper, salt, tomato sauce, cheddar cheese, and pepperoni. Blend the ingredients, apart from cheese and tomato sauce, to make a thick mixture. Heat the waffle iron, pour half the mixture, and cook. Pour tomato sauce and add cheese over the waffles. Broil for 4-5 minutes in oven, and add pepperoni on top.

Lunch- Mixed Veg Zoodles

Yields	:	2- 3
Preparation time	:	5 min
Total time	:	15-20 min

Ingredients:

Butter	1 tablespoon
Olive oil	2 tablespoon
Garlic olive oil	1 tablespoon
Red pepper flakes	½ tablespoon

Minced Garlic	½ tablespoon
Zucchini noodles	3 cups
Parmesan cheese	1.5 cups
Basil	as per taste
Asiago cheese	½ cup

Directions:

Melt butter in a non- stick frying pan and add garlic olive oil. Add red pepper flakes, garlic, red pepper (chopped), and sauté for a minute. Add zucchini noodles and stir for 1-2 minutes. Switch off the heat, toss with grated parmaesan and basil. Take out the zoodles in a bowl, top using asiago cheese, and serve.

Dinner- Cheeseburger Bacon Casserole

Yields	:	2- 3
Preparation time	:	30 min
Total time	:	45 min

Ingredients:

Ground beef	1 pound
Bacon slices	3
Almond flour	½ cup
Riced Cauliflower	3 cups
Husk powder	1 tablespoon
Garlic powder	½ teaspoon
Onion powder	½ teaspoon
Reduced sugar ketchup	2 tablespoons
Dijon mustard	1 tablespoon
Mayo	2 tablespoon
Eggs	3 large
Cheddar cheese	4 ounces
Salt	as per taste
Pepper	as per taste

Directions:

Collect ground beef, bacon slices, almond four, cauliflower, husk powder, garlic powder, onion powder, reduced sugar ketchup, Dijon mustard, mayonnaise, eggs, cheddar cheese, pepper, and salt. Make cauliflower rice in a food processor.

Combine it with dry ingredients, bacon slices, and ground beef to make a crumbly paste. Put the mixture in a frying pan over high medium heat, and season it with pepper and salt. Shred cheese over the meat. Take it out in a bowl. Add shredded cheddar cheese. Now, put ketchup, mayo, mustard, and eggs in the mixture and combine it using fork. Put the mixture into a baking dish lined using parchment paper. Top it with some more cheddar cheese. Bake it in a preheated oven at 350F for 30 minutes. Take out, let cool and serve.

Day 8

Breakfast- Keto Pepperjack Burgers

Yields   :   2- 3
Preparation time :   25 min
Total time   :   35 min

Ingredients:

Sausage	4 ounce
Pepperjack cheese	2 ounces
Bacon	4 slices
Eggs	2 large
Butter	1 tablespoon
Peanut butter powder	1 tablespoon
Pepper	as per taste
Salt	as per taste

Directions:

Collect sausage, pepperjack cheese, bacon, eggs, butter, peanut butter powder, pepper, and salt. Bake the pieces of bacon in the oven for 22-25 minutes at 400F. Combine butter and peanut butter powder. Make sausages and cook them in a pan. Add cheese, cover the pan with a cover, and take it off the heat. Take out the patties and cook an egg in the pan. Assemble the burger and serve.

Lunch- Balsamic Zoodle Strawberry Salad

Yields	:	2- 3
Preparation time	:	10 min
Total time	:	15 min

Ingredients for salad:

Zucchini noodles	1 cup
Sliced Strawberry	1
Goat cheese (herbed)	1 tablespoon
Pistachios	1 tablespoon

Ingredients for Dressing

Strawberries	4
Balsamic vinegar	2 tablespoon
Avocado oil	2 tablespoon

Minced garlic	½ teaspoon
Cracked pepper	1/8 teaspoon
Salt	1/8 teaspoon

Directions:

Collect zucchini noodles, strawberry, goat cheese (herbed), and pistachios for the salad. Gather strawberries, balsamic vinegar, avocado oil, minced garlic, cracked pepper, and salt for dressing. Toss the ingredients of salad in a bowl. Blend the ingredients of dressing and mix the amount you want into the salad. Enjoy the salad.

Dinner- Chicken Nacho Casserole

Yields	:	2- 3
Preparation time	:	20 min
Total time	:	30 min

Ingredients:

| Chili seasoning | 1.5 teaspoon |
| Pepper | as per taste |

Salt	as per taste
Olive oil	2 tablespoon
Sour cream	¼ cup
Cream cheese	4 ounces
Cheddar cheese	4 ounces
Chicken	1.75 pounds
Tomatoes & Green chilies	1 cup
Parmesan cheese	3 tablespoon
Cauliflower	16 ounce- pack
Jalapeno pepper chunk	1 medium
Cilantro	for dressing

Directions:

Season small pieces of chicken with chili seasoning, pepper, and salt, and cook them in olive oil over high medium heat to brown them. Add sour cream, cream cheese, and shredded cheddar cheese, and stir well. Transfer the chicken to a casserole dish. Cook frozen cauliflower in a microwave to cook through. Add cheddar cheese and blend it with an immersion blender. Season with pepper and salt and spread the mixture in a casserole dish. Sprinkle jalapeno chunks and bake in a preheated oven at 375F for 15-20 minutes. Garnish with cilantro and serve.

Day 9

Breakfast- Cheddar Jalapeno Waffles

Yields	:	2- 3
Preparation time	:	10 min
Total time	:	20 min

Ingredients:

Cream cheese	3 ounces
Eggs	3 large
Coconut flour	1 tablespoon
Husk powder	1 teaspoon
Baking powder	1 teaspoon
Cheddar cheese	1 ounce
Jalapeno	1 small
Pepper	as per taste
Salt	as per taste
Toppings of your choice	

Directions:

Collect cream cheese, eggs, coconut flour, husk powder, baking powder, cheddar cheese, jalapeno, pepper, and salt. Blend all the ingredients in a blender and make a smooth paste. Heat the waffle iron, and pour the mixture. Cook for 5-6 minutes. Use your favorite toppings on the top and serve.

Lunch- Sundried Tomato Goat Cheese Orbs

Yields	:	2- 3
Preparation time	:	5 min
Total time	:	10 min

Ingredients:

Sundried Tomato Goat cheese	1 pack of 4 ounces
De-shelled pistachios	½ cup
Salt	as per taste
Pistachios	as per taste

Directions:

Collect sundried tomato, goat cheese, shelled pistachios, and salt. Cut the cheese into a few slices and make balls from them. Crush the pistachios with mortar and pestle. Add salt into this mixture and roll the balls to cover them with pistachios. Roll once more and enjoy.

Dinner- Chicken with Vegetables

Yields	:	2- 3
Preparation time	:	10 min
Total time	:	30 min

Ingredients for rice:

Boned chicken thighs	2 medium
Ground ginger	1 teaspoon
Pepper	as per taste
Salt	as per taste
Peanuts	¼ cups
Green pepper	½ medium
Spring onions	2 large
Deseeded bird eye chili	4 red

Ingredients for sauce:

Soy sauce	1 tablespoon
Rice wine vinegar	2 teaspoon
Chili garlic paste	2 tablespoon
Reduced sugar ketchup	1 tablespoon
Sesame oil	2 teaspoon
Maple syrup	½ teaspoon
Liquid stevia	10 drops

Directions:

For making rice, collect boned chicken thighs, ground ginger, pepper, salt, peanuts, green pepper, spring onions, deseeded Bird Eye Chili. For making sauce, collect soy sauce, rice wine vinegar, chili garlic paste, reduced sugar ketchup, sesame oil, maple syrup, and liquid stevia. Debone the chicken, cut it into small pieces, and season with ground ginger, pepper, and salt. Add chicken in a heated pan and brown it. Chop the vegetables. Make the ketchup by blending all the ingredients of ketchup. After chicken is ready, stir it well and let cook. After 5 minutes, add peanuts and vegetables to cook for 3-4 minutes. Pour the ketchup to boil. Take out and serve.

Day 10

Breakfast- Pancake Doughnuts

Yields	:	2- 3
Preparation time	:	10 min
Total time	:	15 min

Ingredients:

Cream cheese	3 ounce
Eggs	3 large
Almond flour	4 tablespoon
Coconut flour	1 tablespoon
Baking powder	1 teaspoon
Vanilla extract	1 teaspoon
Erythritol	4 tablespoon
Liquid stevia	10 drops

Directions:

Collect cream cheese, eggs, almond flour, coconut flour, baking powder, vanilla extract, erythritol, and liquid stevia.

Blend these ingredients in a bowl. Heat up the doughnut maker and spray it using coconut oil. Now, pour the batter into the wells of donut maker. Cook them for 3 minutes per side and then flip it over. Cook for 2 minutes and then take out the donuts. Let cool and serve.

Lunch- Deviled Salad Eggs

Yields	:	2- 3
Preparation time	:	10 min
Total time	:	15 min

Ingredients:

Eggs	6 large
Chopped chicken	1 cup
Mayonnaise	2 tablespoon
Dijon mustard	1 teaspoon
Chopped onions	1 tablespoon
Celery salt	1 pinch
Dill	½ teaspoon
Pepper lemon seasoning	½ teaspoon

Old bay seasoning   as per taste

Directions:

Collect eggs, chopped chicken, mayonnaise, Dijon mustard, chopped onions, celery salt, dill, pepper lemon seasoning, and old bay seasoning. Combine all the ingredients, leaving aside eggs. Refrigerate the salad. Boil the eggs, shell them, let cool, and half them. Take out the yolks. You can either mix them with the salad or eat separately. Fill the eggs with the chicken salad. Sprinkle old bay seasoning and serve.

Dinner- Kentucky Burgoo

Yields	:	2- 3
Preparation time	:	20 hours
Total time	:	21 hours

Ingredients:

Pot roast	2 pounds for dinner, 2 pounds for burgoo
Beef broth	2 cups
Thyme	1 teaspoon

Celery salt	¼ teaspoon
Basil	1 teaspoon
Dried dill weed	2 teaspoon
Garlic powder	2 teaspoon
Garlic salt	1 teaspoon
Oregano	1 tablespoon
Powdered buttermilk	1 tablespoon
Onion powder	1 tablespoon, 2 teaspoon
Dried parsley	1 tablespoon, 2 teaspoon

Directions:

Collect these dry ingredients- pot roast for dinner and burgoo, beef broth, thyme, celery salt, basil, dried dill weed, garlic powder, pepper, garlic salt, oregano, powdered buttermilk, onion powder, and dried parsley. Set the crock-pot to low and add beef broth and pot roast. Make a mix of dried ingredients and rub it on the pot roast. Cook for 6-8 hours. Boil one large chicken breast for 40 minutes, shred it, and refrigerate it. Open the crock-pot when chicken is ready. Add chicken breast, chili and tomato mixture, diced tomatoes, minced garlic, polish kielbasa, chicken stock, pepper flakes, hot sauce, and chopped onion. Cook for 12-20 hours. Serve.

Day 11

Breakfast- Chive Cheddar Omelet

Yields	:	2- 3
Preparation time	:	10 min
Total time	:	15 min

Ingredients:

Bacon	2 slices
Bacon fat	1 teaspoon
Eggs	2 large
Cheddar cheese	1 ounce
Chives	2 stalks
Pepper	as per taste
Salt	as per taste

Directions:

Collect cooked bacon, eggs, cheddar cheese, chives, pepper, and salt. Prepare all the ingredients and heat a frying pan on low- medium heat with bacon fat. Add eggs; season them with salt, pepper, and chives. After the edges of the omelet are set, add bacon in the middle and cook for at least 20-30 seconds. Switch off the heat and add cheese over the bacon. Fold the edges over the cheese as you do in a burrito. Use cheese as glue to stick the edges in place. Flip to the other side and warm. Serve.

Lunch- Meat Croquettes

Yields	:	2- 3
Preparation time	:	50 min
Total time	:	60 min

Ingredients:

Ground beef	1 pound
Ground pork	1 pound
Whiskey bacon caramelized onions	1 cup
Goat cheese	8 ounces
Onion powder	1 teaspoon
Garlic powder	1 teaspoon
Cinnamon	½ teaspoon

Directions:

Collect ground beef, ground pork, onions, whiskey, bacon grease, goat cheese, onion powder, garlic powder, and cinnamon. Heat bacon grease over medium heat, add sliced onions, and cook for 5-6 minutes. Chop the onions with a wooden spatula. Cook for 20 minutes, add whiskey and water. Combine the ingredients in a bowl, keeping aside goat cheese. Make balls from this mixture, create a pocket in them, and add goat cheese into the pockets. Cover the balls with residual mixture of burger and flatten. Bake the croquettes in a preheated oven at 400F for 30 minutes. Swap to broil after the temperature is reached. Take out and serve.

Dinner- Loaded Banana Peppers

Yields	:	2- 3
Preparation time	:	35 min
Total time	:	45 min

Ingredients:

Garlic olive oil   1 tablespoon

Chopped Banana peppers	2-3
Sweet sausage	2
Ghee	2 tablespoon
Herbs mix	as per taste
Chopped onions	3 tablespoon
Marinara sauce	3 tablespoon
Mozzarella cheese	1.5 cups
Tomato sauce	1/3 cup
Parmesan cheese	as per taste
Italian seasoning	as per taste

Directions:

Collect banana peppers, sweet sausage, ghee, herbs mix, chopped onions, and marinara sauce. Rub olive oil over banana peppers and bake them in a preheated oven at 350F for 20 minutes. Cook sausage over medium heat to crumble them. Add ghee, onions, and herbs mix, and cook on simmer for 5 minutes. Take out the banana peppers and raise the broiler upto 500. Stuff the banana peppers with the mixture of sausage. Top it using mozzarella cheese. Now, place banana peppers onto cookie dish. Pour a coating of marinara, cook for 10 minutes to bubble mozzarella. Serve.

Day 12

Breakfast- Chive Cheddar Omelet

Yields	:	2- 3
Preparation time	:	10 min
Total time	:	15 min

Ingredients:

Bacon	2 slices
Eggs	1 teaspoon
Cheddar cheese	1 ounce
Chives	2 stalks
Pepper	as per taste
Salt	as per taste

Directions:

Collect cooked bacon, eggs, cheddar cheese, chives, pepper, and salt. Prepare all the ingredients and heat a frying pan on low- medium heat with bacon fat. Add eggs; season them with salt, pepper, and chives. After the edges of the omelet are set, add bacon in the middle and cook for at least 20-30 seconds.

Switch off the heat and add cheese over the bacon. Fold the edges over the cheese as you do in a burrito. Use cheese as glue to stick the edges in place. Flip to the other side and warm. Serve.

Lunch- Thyme Lemon Chicken

Yields	:	2- 3
Preparation time	:	40 min
Total time	:	60 min + 1 hour (for soaking the skewers)

Ingredients:

Rosemary skewers	10 skewers of 6 inches each
Tenderloins	1.5 pounds
Fresh thyme	few sprigs
Garlic salt	½ tablespoon
Pepper lemon seasoning	½ tablespoon
Rosemary olive oil	½ tablespoon

Directions:

Gather rosemary skewers, tenderloins, fresh thyme, garlic salt, pepper lemon seasoning, and rosemary olive oil. Soak the skewers in water for 1-2 hours. Sharpen the ends of the skewers using a sharp knife. Toss the chicken pieces in the mixture of remaining ingredients. Slither the leaves off from thyme sprigs, sprinkle them onto the chicken, and skewer the pieces onto the rosemary sticks. Bake them in a preheated oven for 40 minutes at 350F.

Dinner- Banana Pepper Pizza

Yields	:	2- 3
Preparation time	:	15 min
Total time	:	20 min

Ingredients:

Garlic Olive oil	1 tablespoon
Mozzarella	1.5 cups
Tomato sauce	1/3 cup
Grated cheese	as per taste
Pizza seasoning	as per taste

Toppings:

Chopped Banana peppers
Chopped yellow Onions

Directions:

Heat garlic with oil in a non-stick ceramic pan, add mozzarella, and spread it evenly. Cook for 4-5 minutes to make it crisp on the edges. Spread tomato sauce on the pizza base in the pan and cook for a minute. Using a wooden ladle, take off the crust from the pan and place it on an even surface. Sprinkle grated cheese, pizza seasonings, and top it with sausage, mozzarella, banana peppers, and onions. Place it in a preheated oven at 500F for two minutes to heat up the toppings. Let cool for two minutes to settle the cheese. Serve in pieces.

Day 13

Breakfast- Keto Cream and Berries Cake

Yields	:	2- 3
Preparation time	:	20 min
Total time	:	25 min

Ingredients:

Vanilla bean sugar free sweetener	¼ cup
Eggs	2 large
Ghee	2 tablespoon
Almond flour	¼ cup
Organic cream cheese	2 tablespoon
Mixed Berries	¼ cup

Whipped cream:

Heavy cream	¼ cup
Brown sugar	½tablespoon

Directions:

Take a bowl and blend sweetener, eggs, cream cheese, and ghee to make a smooth mixture. Take out the mixture in a microwave safe dish. Add almond flour, stir, and then stir the berries. Now, microwave this batter for 4 minutes on high. Put the brown sugar and heavy cream on a single serve blender and blend to make a stiff mixture. After the cake is ready, let it cool and add up whipped cream. Enjoy.

Lunch- Cheese and Dijon Steak

Yields	:	2- 3
Preparation time	:	10 min
Total time	:	15 min

Ingredients:

Ghee	1 tablespoon
Chopped Onions	¼ cup
Minced Garlic	1 tablespoon
Green peppers	¼ cup
Olive oil	1 tablespoon

Shaved steak	1 pound
Dijon mix	as per taste
Mayo	2 tablespoon
American cheese	4 slices

Directions:

Heat ghee in a non- stick frying pan, add onions, garlic, and green peppers, and sauté them. Pour olive oil, then shaved steak, and cook to brown them. Simmer the heat. Add Dijon mix and mayonnaise. Put American cheese over the steak and cook for 60 seconds. Mix well to melt the cheese. Take out in a bowl and serve.

Dinner- Pea Pods with Coconut

Yields	:	2- 3
Preparation time	:	10 min
Total time	:	15 min

Ingredients:

Salted Butter	4 tablespoon

Coconut oil	1 tablespoon
Shredded coconut	½ cup
Cinnamon	½ teaspoon
Rosemary	1 tablespoon
Chopped pea pods	7 ounces
Salt	as per taste

Directions:

Melt butter in a pan over low medium heat and add coconut oil. Add shredded coconut and coat it with fat. Add cinnamon and rosemary oil and combine. Simmer the heat and cook for a minute. Add broadly chopped up pea pods in the mixture and mix. Slightly raise the flame and cook for 5 minutes. Sprinkle salt and mix.

Day 14

Breakfast-Cauli Cajun Hash

Yields	:	2- 3
Preparation time	:	10 min
Total time	:	20 min

Ingredients:

Chopped onions	¼ onion
Minced garlic	2 tablespoon
Chopped and steamed cauliflower	1 pound bag
Cajun seasoning	1 teaspoon
Chopped green peppers	½
Red Pastrami	8 ounce
Egg	1

Directions:

Sauté chopped onions in olive oil over medium heat, and sauté garlic after the onions become transparent. Drain excess water from chopped and steamed cauliflower. Add the cauliflower to the onions and sauté for 8-10 minutes to brown them. Mix

Cajun seasoning, add chopped green peppers and pastrami. Toss the ingredients. Take out the mixture in bowls. Now cook an egg with sunny side up, and add it over the top of mixture in bowls. Add Cajun seasoning and serve.

Lunch- Egg Avocado Salad

Yields	:	1
Preparation time	:	5 min
Total time	:	10 min

Ingredients:

Boiled eggs	1 large
Spicy guacamole	2 teaspoon
Mayonnaise	1 teaspoon
Pepper	as per taste
Salt	as per taste
Chunks of avocado	½ cup

Directions:

Collect hard- boiled egg, avocado chunks, spicy guacamole, mayonnaise, pepper, and salt. Dice the eggs with the help of an egg slicer. Combine the ingredients of salad, add pepper and salt, and combine them with eggs. Serve.

Dinner- Salad with Brussels Sprouts and Cheese

Yields	:	2
Preparation time	:	5 min
Total time	:	10 min

Ingredients:

Brussels sprouts	6
Olive oil	1 teaspoon
Apple cider vinegar	½ teaspoon
Pepper	as per taste
Salt	as per taste
Parmesan cheese	1 tablespoon

| Lemon juice | ½ teaspoon |

Directions:

Wash and dry Brussels sprouts, cut them in half till the roots. Cut slim slices, and toss them in a bowl. Add oil, apple cider, pepper, salt, and mix. Sprinkle parmesan cheese and serve. You can also sprinkle lemon juice.

Day 15

Breakfast- Low Carb Keto Cereal

Yields	:	2- 3
Preparation time	:	15 min
Total time	:	20 min

Ingredients:

Coconut oil	1 tablespoon
Coconut flakes	1 packet
Cinnamon powder	1 teaspoon
Keto cereal	2 cups
Sliced strawberry	½ cup
Dark chocolate roasted almonds	¼ cup
Unsweetened almond milk	1.5 cups

Directions:

Grease the cookie sheet using coconut oil and pour coconut flakes over the cookie sheet to make a layer. Bake in the preheated oven at 350 degrees for 5 minutes. Keep a watch, jumble up the flakes, let them toast and tan. Pull out the dish and sprinkle cinnamon powder, add keto cereal, sliced strawberry, dark chocolate roasted almonds, and unsweetened almond milk. Serve.

Lunch- Tuna Dill Salad Sandwich

Yields	:	2- 3
Preparation time	:	10 min
Total time	:	30 min

Ingredients:

Tuna	1 can
Mayonnaise	3 tablespoon
Dried dill	1 pinch
Pepper	as per taste
Salt	as per taste
Hamburger dills	5-6
Skewers	

Directions:

Gather tuna, mayonnaise, dried dill, pepper, salt, and hamburger dills. Combine the ingredients, leaving aside the pickles, and refrigerate it for 30 minutes. Stick the mixture between two hamburger chips, secure them with a skewer, and serve.

Dinner- Chicken Soup with Cream

Yields	:	2- 3
Preparation time	:	20 min
Total time	:	30 min

Ingredients:

Halves of Chicken breasts	3-4
Water	3.5 quarts
Diced onion	1
Italian seasoning	2 teaspoon
Sliced lemon	½ lemon
Minced garlic	3
Bay leaves	2
Bouillon cubes, chicken	4
Pepper	as per taste

Salt	as per taste
Chardonnay	2/3 cup
Chopped parsley	3 tablespoon
Chopped rosemary	2 teaspoon
Heavy cream	¾ cup
Grated parmesan	1 cup

Directions:

Collect halves of chicken breasts, water, diced onion, Italian seasoning, sliced lemon, minced garlic, bay leaves, bouillon cubes, pepper, and salt for broth. Keep chardonnay, chopped rosemary, heavy cream, grated parmesan, and heavy cream for further steps. Take a deep pot and pour all the ingredients. Cook chicken up to a temperature of 180 degrees. Take it out of the soup, let cool, and shred it. Strain the soup into a large vessel and discard the rest. Pour it back to the pot. Add the remaining ingredients and cook on low for 10 minutes. Add shredded chicken and cook for 5 minutes. Serve.

Day 16

Breakfast- Pumpkin Cheese Pancakes

Yields	:	2- 3
Preparation time	:	5 min
Total time	:	10 min

Ingredients for pumpkin butter:

100% Pumpkin	½ tablespoon
Butter	3 tablespoon
Stevia	1/16 teaspoon

Ingredients for pancakes:

Eggs	2
Pumpkin pie spice	¼ tablespoon
Coconut flour	2 tablespoon
Cream cheese	2 ounces

Directions:

Mix pumpkin and butter and microwave the mixture at intervals of 10 seconds to make a smooth mixture. Add Stevia as you like. Now, blend eggs, pumpkin pie spice, coconut flour, and cream cheese. Heat a non-stick frying pan and add butter. When the butter browns, add the batter. Flip it after the bubbles arise and cook for 50-60 seconds. Take off the heat, top it with pumpkin butter, and serve.

Lunch- Chicken Wings

Yields	:	2- 3
Preparation time	:	40 min
Total time	:	50 min

Ingredients:

Frozen wings	20
Garlic salt	1 teaspoon
Garlic olive oil	2 tablespoon
Grated parmesan	1 cup
Garlic powder	½ tablespoon

Directions:

Gather frozen wings, garlic salt, garlic olive oil, grated Parmesan, and garlic powder. Arrange the frozen wings over a roasting rack placed onto a baking pan. Sprinkle garlic salt, and bake them in a preheated oven at 450F for 30 minutes in a preheated oven at 450F. Add garlic oil and cook on broil for 5 minutes so that the skin becomes crispy and brown. Take the chicken out of the oven, toss them in a bowl, coat with another layer of garlic oil. Sprinkle garlic powder and serve.

Dinner- Garlic Pasta with Yellow Squash

Yields	:	2- 3
Preparation time	:	10 min
Total time	:	15 min

Ingredients:

Summer squash	3
Pepper lemon seasoning	as per taste
Olive oil	2 tablespoon
Chopped parsley	½ cup

Garlic	1 teaspoon
Chopped Almonds	1/3 cup
Salt	as per taste
Lemon juice	½ lemon
Keto pasta	

Directions:

Remove the end of summer squash, and peel them. When the seeds are visible, stop peeling. Toss the strips of squash in a bowl with pepper lemon seasoning. Put olive oil in a cast iron skillet and heat it over high medium flame for a while. Add chopped parsley, garlic, and almonds. Add chopped summer squash and cook for 2 minute. Switch off the flame, add salt, and toss the ingredients. Squeeze lemon over keto pasta. Serve.

Day 17

Breakfast- Low Carb Pancakes

Yields   :   2- 3
Preparation time :
Total time   :

Ingredients:

Cream cheese	2 ounce
Eggs	2
Cinnamon powder	½ teaspoon
Coconut flour	1 tablespoon
Stevia	½ packet
Coconut oil	1 tablespoon
Salted butter	½ teaspoon
Maple syrup	½ teaspoon
Butter	½ tablespoon

Directions:

Collect cream cheese, eggs, cinnamon powder, coconut flour, and Stevia. Blend all the ingredients to make a smooth mixture. Heat a skillet or non-stick frying pan and add coconut oil or salted butter over medium high heat. Pour the batter to make pancakes. Flip it over to cook on the other side. Top it with maple syrup (sugar free), or butter. Serve.

Lunch- Caesar salad

Yields	:	2- 3
Preparation time	:	15 min
Total time	:	20 min

Ingredients:

Egg yolk	1
Dijon Mustard	1 teaspoon
Avocado oil	8 tablespoon
Anchovies filets	4
Apple cider vinegar	3 tablespoon
Minced Garlic cloves	4
Romaine leaves	24 whole
Pork coated croutons	2 ounce
Shaved parmesan	4 tablespoon

Directions:

Blend egg yolk, mustard, ACV, and pulse. Carefully pour avocado oil over the mixture and blend on low. Mayonnaise will form from the combination of egg yolk and oil. You can also use ready mayo. Add anchovies, grated parmesan, and garlic, and blend on low to make a smooth mayo like dressing. Clean, wash, dry your romaine leaves, place them on serving plates, and spread the dressing onto them. Put a few pieces of pork-coated croutons and garnish using shaved parmesan.

Dinner- Steak Stuffed Green Bell Peppers

Yields	:	2- 3
Preparation time	:	30 min
Total time	:	45 min

Ingredients:

Green peppers	4
Chopped Onion	¼ cup
Butter	1 tablespoon
Mayonnaise	2 tablespoon

Garlic	1 teaspoon
Shaved steak	1 pound
Montreal steak seasoning	as per taste
Cheese slice	7 slices

Directions:

Cut the green peppers from the top and bake them in a preheated oven at 400F. Chop the green peppers tops, onions, butter, and garlic, and heat them in a frying pan to soften. Put shaved steak and sprinkle Montreal steak. Mix well and chop the mixture with spatula. Take out the green peppers from oven. Add a cheese slice to the frying pan to melt it. Turn off the heat. Place half cheese slice in each bell pepper, and spoon the mixture into the shells of peppers. Add a cheese slice on the top, and bake it for 5 minutes to melt the cheese.

Day 18

Breakfast- Egg Porridge

Yields	:	2- 3
Preparation time	:	10 min
Total time	:	15 min

Ingredients:

Sweetener	2 tablespoon
Organic Eggs	2
Heavy cream	1/3 cup
Butter	2 tablespoon
Cinnamon	1/8 tablespoon

Directions:

Combine cream, sweetener, and eggs in a bowl and whisk them. Heat butter over medium high flame to melt the butter. Add cream mixture and eggs, and cook the eggs so that the mixture thickens. It will start curdling. When you observe the tiny grains, remove the saucepan from the heat. Take out the porridge into a serving bowl. Now, sprinkle cinnamon and serve.

Lunch- Pesto Chicken Salad

Yields   :   2- 3
Preparation time :   10 min
Total time   :   12 min

Ingredients:

Cubed cooked chicken	1 pound
Sliced bacon	6 slices
Avocado	1 medium
Grape tomatoes	10
Mayonnaise	¼ cup
Pesto	2 tablespoon
Leaves of butter lettuce	

Directions:

Gather cubed cooked chicken, sliced bacon, avocado, grape tomatoes, mayonnaise, pesto and leaves of butter lettuce.

Combine the ingredients in a bowl, except lettuce leaves and toss gently. Spread he salad onto the lettuce leaves placed in a bowl and serve.

Dinner- Buffalo Strips

Yields	:	2- 3
Preparation time	:	30 min
Total time	:	35 min

Ingredients:

Pounded Chicken breasts	5
Hot sauce	½ cup
Olive oil	¼ cup
Butter	3 tablespoon
Chili powder	1 tablespoon
Paprika	1 tablespoon
Pepper	as per taste
Salt	as per taste
Onion powder	1 teaspoon
Garlic powder	1 teaspoon

Almond flour	¾ cup
Eggs	3 large
Crumbled blue cheese	3 tablespoon

Directions:

Wash the chicken breasts and pat dry. Flatten them using a meat hammer. Take a ramekin and combine chili powder, paprika, pepper, salt, onion powder, and garlic powder. Combine some spice mix and almond flour in a bowl. Wrap a cookie sheet with aluminum foil and place it over the cooling rack. Season the chicken with the one- third of spice mix on one side. Season the other side with remaining spices. Whisk eggs in a bowl, dip chicken into it, and coat it in almond flour. Place them on cooling rack. Heat butter and hot sauce in a pan over low heat, and bake the chicken in a preheated oven 400F for 15 minutes. Coat it with olive oil and bake for 3 more minutes on each side. Take out, let cool, and serve with crumbled blue cheese and prepared sauce.

Day 19

Breakfast- Buttered Green Eggs

Yields	:	2- 3
Preparation time	:	15 min
Total time	:	20 min

Ingredients:

Coconut oil	1 tablespoon
Butter	2 tablespoon
Chopped garlic	2 cloves
Thyme	1 teaspoon
Parsley	½ cup
Cilantro	½ cup
Eggs	4
Ground cumin	¼ teaspoon
Ground cayenne	¼ teaspoon
Sea salt	½ teaspoon
Breakfast sausage	

Directions:

Melt coconut oil and butter in a non-stick frying pan, and add chopped garlic. Let it cook on low heat for 3 minutes to brown the garlic. Add thyme and cook for 30 seconds. Add parsley and cilantro, and cook for 3 minutes. Crack eggs into the pan, and cover the frying pan using its lid and simmer the heat for 4-6 minutes. The yolks should set while being soft inside. Serve it in a plate with breakfast sausage.

Lunch- Smoked Chicken Salad

Yields	:	2- 3
Preparation time	:	4-5 hours
Total time	:	5 hours 30 min

Ingredients:

Smoked cubed chicken	4 cups
Organic mayonnaise	1 cup
Paprika	1 teaspoon
Chopped onions	1

Sea salt	1 teaspoon
Ground pepper	as per taste
Hard-boiled eggs	1
Chopped celery	1 cup
Shredded green pepper	½ cup
Protein buns	8
Wood chips	

Directions:

Gather smoked cubed chicken, organic mayonnaise, paprika, chopped onions, sea salt, ground pepper, hard- boiled eggs, chopped celery, shredded green pepper, and protein buns. Breakdown and clean the chicken pieces into breasts, wings, and thighs. Position soaked chips of wood at the base of the smoker. Put chicken over the racks and smoke them for 3-4 hours. You can also complete their cooking in a preheated oven at 250F for half an hour.

Combine salt and paprika with mayonnaise. Add other ingredients and chopped smoked chicken. Season with pepper and salt, add sliced eggs, and refrigerate for an hour. Take out and serve with protein buns to shape sandwiches.

Dinner- Pancakes with Blueberries

Yields	:	2- 3
Preparation time	:	10 min
Total time	:	15 min

Ingredients:

Cream cheese	4 ounces
Eggs	4
Granulated brown sugar	2 tablespoon
Cinnamon	1 dash
Maple syrup	½ teaspoon
Fresh blueberries or strawberries	

Directions:

Blend cream cheese, eggs, granulated brown sugar, and cinnamon with an immersion blender to make a smooth mixture. Let it sit for 2 minutes to settle the bubbles. Pour some batter into a heated pan coated with butter. Cook on one side for 2 minutes and for 1 minute on the other side. Serve with maple syrup and fresh blueberries or strawberries.

Day 20

Breakfast- Chive and Cheddar Soufflés

Yields   :   2- 3

Preparation time   :   25 min

Total time   :   40 min

Ingredients:

Ingredient	Amount
Almond flour	½ cup
Ground Mustard	1 teaspoon
Salt	1 teaspoon
Pepper	½ teaspoon
Xanthan gum	½ teaspoon
Heavy cream	¾ cup
Cayenne pepper	¼ teaspoon
Whisked chives	¼ cup
Egg yolks	6
Cheddar Cheese	2 cups
Cream of tartar	¼ teaspoon

Directions:

Grease the ramekins (6-8 ounce) and set them on a cookie sheet. Combine almond flour, mustard, salt, pepper, xanthan, cayenne, and gum, and whisk all the ingredients. Now, add and whisk chives, egg yolks, and cheese. Take a separate bowl and beat the egg white along with salt and cream of tartar to make a glossy mixture. Now, divide this mixture into the ramekins, place the cookie sheet in the preheated oven, and bake for 25 minutes so that the soufflés rise to an inch above the edge and become golden brown. Serve hot.

Lunch- Chimichurri Salad and Steak

Yields	:	2- 3
Preparation time	:	10 min
Total time	:	15 min

Ingredients:

Shredded romaine hearts	2 cups
Shredded red cabbage	1/3 cup
Thinly sliced radishes	2

Coarsely chopped cilantro	2 tablespoon
Salad dressing	1 tablespoon
Chimichurri sauce	3 tablespoon
Great steak	4 ounces
Blue cheese	1 ounce

Directions:

Gather shredded romaine hearts, shredded red cabbage, thinly sliced radishes, coarsely chopped cilantro, salad dressing, chimichurri sauce, and great steak for salad, and blue cheese for topping. Combine romaine hearts, red cabbage, radishes, cilantro, and salad dressing in a bowl. Grill the steak and place it aside the salad with chimichurri sauce to dip. Crumble blue cheese over the salad. Serve.

Dinner- Fried Chicken

Yields	:	2- 3
Preparation time	:	10 min
Total time	:	20 min + 1 night for refrigerating

Ingredients:

Chicken breasts	3 large
Egg	2 whole
Crumbled pork rinds	4 ounces
Peanut oil	2 cups
Dip of your choice	

Directions:

Put pickle juice and chicken breasts in a zip lock freezer bag and refrigerate overnight. Drain the juices from the bag and make nuggets of the chicken. Coat the chicken in egg and then in crumbled pork rinds. Heat peanut oil in a medium frying pan and fry chicken pieces on each side for 2-3 minutes. Take them out on a paper towel and serve with your favorite dip.

Day 21

Breakfast- Eggs Benedict

Yields	:	2- 3
Preparation time	:	
Total time	:	

Ingredients:

Egg whites and Egg yolks	3
Mix herbs	2 tablespoons
Water	
Lemon juice	½ lemon
Dijon Mustard sauce	2 tablespoon
Butter	1.5 cups
Cayenne Pepper	1/8 teaspoon
Salt	½ teaspoon

Directions:

Whip the egg whites separately, mix herbs, protein powder, and reserve. Now, fold the eggs yolks to this mixture. Pour this mixture into the greased cookie sheet to make hamburgers, and bake for 30 minutes. Let cool entirely. To make the sauce, boil 1 inch height of water in a flat saucepan, and simmer. Put lemon juice, egg yolks, mustard in the double boiler. Whisk the yolk mixture and blend. Add butter steadily, cook, and whisk. Add pepper, cayenne, salt, and continue to whisk. Now, place the bun halves on the plate, top them with ham.

To poach the eggs, boil 1 inch height of water in a wide pan and simmer. Crack eggs in water gently, one by one. Use slotted spoon to take out the eggs, pat dry, and place them over ham. Top them with the sauce. Serve.

Lunch- Keto Pitas

Yields   :   2- 3

Preparation time   :   30 min

Total time   :   35 min

Ingredients:

Coconut flour	7/8 cup
Husk powder	4 tablespoon
Almond flour	2 tablespoon
Coconut oil	½ cup
Dry spices	½ teaspoon
Bone broth	2 cups
Salt	¼ teaspoon
Sweetener	1 teaspoon

Directions:

Collect coconut flour, husk powder, almond flour, coconut oil, dry spices, bone broth, salt, and sweetener like erythritol. Mix the dry ingredients mentioned in a bowl, and whisk well. Add fat, stir well to make a smooth mixture. Pour the hot bone broth, blend evenly, and puff up the dough. Make balls of this dough and flatten them on a parchment sheet. Use rolling pin to make flatbreads. Grease a flat pan with fat or oil and heat it. put the pita on the frying pan and brown its bottom. When one side is cooked through, flip it over. When the bread puffs and bubbles up, after 5-10 minutes take out on a plate. Serve or refrigerate.

Dinner- Daikon Fries

Yields	:	2- 3
Preparation time	:	20 min
Total time	:	30 min

Ingredients:

Diakon radishes	1
Coconut oil	¼ cup
Pepper	as per taste
Salt	as per taste
Seasonings	½ teaspoon
Chipotle mayo	for dipping

Directions:

Wash, peel, and cut diakon radishes into the shape of French Fries. Drain them under a stream of cold water to remove the starch. Pat dry the radishes. Combine coconut oil, pepper, salt, and other seasonings, and cover the radishes with this mixture. Place them on a baking sheet and bake them in a preheated oven at 475F for 15 minutes. Flip them over and bake for 15 more minutes. Take out, let cool, and serve with chipotle mayo.

Day 22

Breakfast- Salmon Avocado Breakfast

Yields   :   1

Preparation time :   5 min

Total time   :   5 min

Ingredients:

Ripe avocado	1
Smoked salmon	2 ounces
Goat cheese	1 ounce
Extra virgin olive oil	2 tablespoon
Lemon	1
Sea salt	a pinch

Directions:

Collect avocado, smoked salmon, goat cheese, olive oil, lemon, and sea salt. Cut avocados and remove seeds. Blend the remaining ingredients to chop them coarsely. Put the cream in the pitted avocados and serve fresh. You can also chop the avocado and salmon in chunks and mix them with the remaining ingredients.

Lunch- Meat Muffins

Yields	: 2- 3
Preparation time	: 15 min
Total time	: 1 hour

Ingredients:

Mushrooms	½ pound
Egg yolks	6
Ground beef	1 pound
Coconut Aminos	2 tablespoon
Coconut flour	¾ cup
Sea salt	1 teaspoon

Directions:

Collect mushrooms, egg yolks, ground beef, coconut Aminos, coconut flour, and sea salt. Chop mushrooms in a food processor; add egg yolks, coconut aminos, and salt, and process to make a smooth puree. Take out the mixture into a bowl, add ground beef, and combine well. Add coconut flour to make soft dough. Place doubled paper cupcakes on a cookie sheet. Make a few meatballs from the dough and put them in the cupcakes. Bake them in a preheated oven at 350F for 45 minutes. Serve hot or cold.

Dinner- Burger with Cheese

Yields	:	2- 3
Preparation time	:	15 min
Total time	:	25 min

Ingredients:

Ground beef	28 ounces
Chopped bacon	8 slices
Cheddar cheese	¼ cup
Minced garlic	2 teaspoon
Black pepper	2 teaspoon
Soy sauce	1 tablespoon

Salt	1.25 teaspoon
Onion powder	1 teaspoon
Worcestershire sauce	1 teaspoon

Directions:

Cook chopped bacon slices in a cast iron skillet, and season them with spices, and cover with grease catcher. After bacon is ready, take it out on paper towels. In a large bowl, combine ground beef, bacon, chopped chives, minced garlic, black pepper, soy sauce, salt, onion powder, and Worcestershire sauce, and mix well. Make patties from this mixture. Pour bacon fat in an iron skillet and fry the patties in hot fat for 3-5 minutes on each side. Serve with onion, cheese and pour Sriracha.

Day 23

Breakfast- Ricotta Pie and Swiss Chard

Yields	:	24muffins
Preparation time	:	35 min
Total time	:	45 min

Ingredients:

Olive oil	1 tablespoon
Chopped onion	½ cup
Minced garlic	1 clove
Chopped Swiss chard	8 cups
Ricotta cheese, whole milk	2 cups
Shredded mozzarella	1 cup
Shredded parmesan	¼ cup
Ground nutmeg	1/8 teaspoon
Salt	as per taste
Pepper	as per taste
Mild sausage	1 pound

Directions:

Sauté garlic and onions in olive oil in a sauce pan. Add Swiss chard and cook to wilt the leaves and soften the stems. Add nutmeg, pepper, and salt. Take off the pan from heat and let cool. Take a bowl and beat a few eggs. Add parmesan, ricotta, and mozzarella. Stir the mixture into the pan. Make pies in a baking sheet and bake in a preheated oven at 350 degrees for 35 minutes.

Lunch- Egg Muffins

Yields	:	2- 3
Preparation time	:	5 min
Total time	:	30 min

Ingredients:

Frozen spinach	2/3 cup
Pesto	3 tablespoon
Pitted olives	½
Sun dried tomatoes	¼ cup

Goat cheese	4.4 ounces
Eggs	6 large
Salt	as per taste
Pepper	as per taste

Directions:

Wash spinach and squeeze excess water, slice and deseed olives, and cut small pieces of sundried tomatoes. Break a few eggs into the bowl, put pesto, and then, season the mixture with pepper and salt. Combine well. Divide the crushed goat cheese, sundried tomatoes, olives, and spinach into muffin pans. Now, pour the mixture into the pan and bake it in a preheated oven at 350F for 20-25 minutes. Take out, let cool and serve.

Dinner- Beer Braised Meatballs

Yields	:	2- 3
Preparation time	:	40 min
Total time	:	1 hour

Ingredients for meatballs:

Ground bison	1 pound
Egg	1
Almond flour	½ cup
Kosher salt	1 teaspoon
Onion powder	1 teaspoon
Allspice	½ teaspoon
Cocoa powder	1 teaspoon
Worcestershire sauce	1 teaspoon
Avocado	1 tablespoon

Ingredients for gravy:

Butter	2 tablespoons
Sliced onions	1 cup
Kosher salt	¼ teaspoon
Ground pepper	1/8 teaspoon
Chocolate stout	1 cup
Sugar substitute	2 tablespoon
Butter	2 tablespoon

Directions:

For making meatballs, collect ground bison, egg, almond flour, kosher salt, ground black pepper, onion powder, allspice, cocoa powder, Worcestershire sauce, Avocado oil to fry. To make gravy, collect butter, sliced onions, salt, pepper, beer broth or chocolate stout, granulated brown sugar and butter. Combine meatball ingredients, leaving aside avocado oil, mix, and make meatballs. Cook them in heated oil for 2-3 minutes on each side to brown properly. Take them out, and put onions and butter into the pan. Cook for 5 minutes, season with pepper, salt, and add sweetener. Put back the meatballs and coat them with onions. Cover with lid and simmer them for 25-30 minutes. Take off the lid and simmer for 5-10 minutes to thicken the gravy. Take meatballs out and serve with parsley garnishing.

Day 24

Breakfast- Low-Carb Fruit Mix

Yields	:	1
Preparation time	:	5 min
Total time	:	5 min

The servings of fruits mentioned below are low in net carbs, and hence, can be taken in breakfast:

Raw strawberries	½ cup
Raw raspberries	½ cup
Medium peach	½ cup
Sweet cherries	5 whole
Kiwi fruit	½
Apricot	1 medium
Haas avocado	½ medium

Lunch- Chicken Liver and Radishes

Yields	:	2- 3

Preparation time	:	5 min
Total time	:	5 min

Ingredients:

Chicken liver	100 grams
Organic butter	3 tablespoon
Chopped herbs	1 teaspoon
Sea salt	a pinch
Ground pepper	as per taste

Directions:

Collect chicken livers, organic butter, chopped thyme, oregano, and sage; sea salt, and freshly ground pepper. Sauté chicken livers. Then, combine all the ingredients into the jar of food processor and pulse to make a smooth paste. Serve with raw crackers or radishes.

Dinner- Pecan Bacon Covered In Chocolate

Yields	:	4-5
Preparation time	:	50 min

Total time   :   60-70 min

Ingredients for bacon base:

Bacon	13 slices
Erythritol	2 tablespoon
Maple extract	1 tablespoon

Ingredients for coating:

Unsweetened cocoa powder	4 tablespoon
Erythritol	2 tablespoon
Liquid stevia	15 drops
Roasted chopped pecans	¼ cup

Directions:

To make bacon base, collect bacon slices, erythritol, and maple extract. To make coating, collect unsweetened cocoa powder, erythritol, liquid stevia, and roasted pecans. Lay the bacon slices in an aluminum foil lined baking sheet. Sprinkle erythritol and maple syrup to rub the bacon on both sides. Bake them in a preheated oven at 400F for 45-50 minutes. Take out, let cool, and take out the bacon fat in a container. In this container, add cocoa powder, erythritol, liquid stevia, and mix. Dip the bacon pieces into this cocoa mixture and transfer them onto a parchment sheet. Sprinkle chopped pecans prior to drying of chocolate. Refrigerate for 5 hours and serve.

Day 25

Breakfast- Onion and Cheese Quiche

Yields	:	2
Preparation time	:	25 min
Total time	:	45 min

Ingredients:

Jack cheese	5-6 cups
Butter	2 tablespoons
Chopped White onion	1 large
Eggs	12 large
Heavy cream	2 cups
Salt	1 teaspoon
Ground pepper	1 teaspoon
Dried thyme	2 teaspoons

Directions:

Melt butter in a skillet over low- medium heat. Sauté chopped onions and take off from heat. Grease two quiche pans and put shredded cheese to make a layer. Add cooled onions in the pan in a layer. Crack a few eggs, add pepper, salt, and thyme, and whisk well. Pour this mixture in the bowl to make a layer. Bake the quiche pans in a preheated oven at 350 degrees for 25 minutes until it becomes puffy. Examine it with the knife test. Serve in pieces.

Lunch- Broccoli Casserole

Yields	:	2- 3
Preparation time	:	50 min
Total time	:	60 min

Ingredients:

Coconut oil	2 tablespoon
Broccoli florets	2 cups
Diced white onion	1 medium
Sea salt	as per taste
Pepper	as per taste
Sliced mushrooms	8 ounces

Directions:

Lubricate a casserole pan using coconut oil. In a separate utensil, steam broccoli and keep aside. Now, heat a saucepan with coconut oil, add onions, pepper, and salt. Add mushrooms and sauté them. Take off the pan from the heat. Transfer broccoli, onions, shredded chicken, and mushrooms into casserole pan. Add bone broth, eggs, nutmeg, coconut oil, pepper, and salt, and blend well. Pour the mixture over the casserole. Bake it in a preheated oven at 350F for 35-40 minutes. Take out, let cool for 5-10 minutes, and serve.

Dinner- Mushroom Alfredo and Celery Chicken

Yields	:	3-4
Preparation time	:	40 min
Total time	:	60 min

Ingredients for noodles:

Celery roots	2 medium
Sea salt	½ teaspoon
Ghee	1 tablespoon

Ingredients for sauce:

Water	¾ cup
Cashews	½ cup
Ghee	1 tablespoon
Lemon juice	1 tablespoon
Onion powder	¼ teaspoon
Garlic powder	¼ teaspoon
Sea salt	¼ teaspoon

Ingredients for mushrooms:

Ghee	1 tablespoon
Chopped mushrooms	3 cup
Sea salt	

Ingredients for chicken:

Ghee	1 teaspoon
Halves of chicken breast	2-4

Onion powder

Salt

Garlic powder

Water   ¼ cup

Directions:

Peel celeriac and spiralize them. Now, sprinkle them with sea salt and heat celery in hot ghee in a pan. Sauté the celery noodles until they reduce to half. Combine water, cashews, ghee, lemon juice, onion powder, garlic powder, and sea salt, and blend them to make sauce. Pour the sauce in the pan, cover it with a lid, slightly cracked. Simmer the heat and cook for 20 minutes. Sauté mushrooms in a different pan in ghee and salt. Rub garlic powder, salt, and onion powder over the chicken pieces and take another pan to cook them for a minute. Add water and cover the chicken pan with a lid, slightly cracked, and simmer the heat for 20 minutes. Chop the chicken into small pieces and add it along with mushrooms to the pan of noodles. Serve with cracked black pepper.

Day 26

Breakfast- Bacon, Onion, and Cheese Quiche

Yields	:	2- 3
Preparation time	:	45 min
Total time	:	60 min

Ingredients:

Bacon slices	
Butter	2 tablespoon
Chopped onions	1 large
Eggs	12
Pepper	1 teaspoon
Salt	1 teaspoon
Thyme	2 teaspoon

Directions:

Place a few bacon slices on the cookie sheet. Bake them in a preheated oven for 20 minutes at 350 degrees. Process them in a food processor once they are cooled. Melt butter in a skillet over low- medium heat. Sauté chopped onions and take off from heat. Grease two quiche pans and put shredded cheese to make a layer. Add cooled onions in the pan in a layer. Crack a few eggs, add pepper, salt, and thyme, and whisk well. Add processed bacon and pour this mixture in the bowl to make a layer. Bake the quiche pans in a preheated oven at 350 degrees for 25 minutes until it becomes puffy. Examine it with the knife test. Serve in pieces.

Lunch- Foiled Juicy Chicken

Yields	:	2- 3
Preparation time	:	10 min
Total time	:	1 hour 40 min

Ingredients:

Chicken breasts with bone	3 pounds
Bouillion beef	1 tablespoon

Granulated garlic	1 tablespoon
Dried onion flakes	2 tablespoon
Freeze dried parsley	1 tablespoon
Ground pepper	as per taste
Tamari, gluten-free	2 tablespoons
Olive oil	2-3 tablespoon

Directions:

Place chicken ribs on a baking pan lined with double layer of aluminum foil. Smear the facing breast sides with bouillon paste. Rub both sides with granulated garlic, ground pepper, and minced onion. Sprinkle tamari, coconut aminos, olive oil, and fermented soy sauce. Now, tightly wrap the pieces of chicken with aluminum foil. Place the pieces on a roasting pan and place it in a preheated oven at 300F for 2 hours. When the chicken temperature reaches 170 degrees in its thickest portion, take out the chicken and remove foil. Save the juices for dipping chicken. Cut the chicken into pieces and pour the juices. Serve.

Dinner- Srirachoy Shrimp Wrapped in Bacon

Yields   :   2- 3
Preparation time :   30 min
Total time   :   50 min

Ingredients:

Frozen shrimp   as many as you want
Bacon slices
Srirachoy suace   ½ cup

Directions:

Dry the precooked frozen shrimps using paper towels. Wrap the shrimps in bacon slices as many as you like and secure them using a toothpick, or just place them with seam facing down on the aluminum foil lined baking sheet. Leave the tails of the shrimp exposed. Use a pastry brush to apply Srirachoy sauce and bake them in a preheated oven for 30 min at 400F. Serve hot.

Day 27

Breakfast- Sausage, Onion and Cheese Quiche

Yields	:	2- 3
Preparation time	:	
Total time	:	

Ingredients:

Chopped onions	1 large
Shredded cheese	5-6 cups
Pork sausage	2-3 ounce
Eggs	12 large
Pepper	as per taste
Salt	as per taste
Thyme	2 teaspoon

Directions:

Melt butter in a skillet over low- medium heat. Sauté chopped onions and take off from heat. Grease two quiche pans and put shredded cheese to make a layer. Add cooled onions in the pan in a layer. Cook pork sausage in a skillet and crumble them. Add a layer of this crumbled sausage to the bowl. Crack a few eggs, add pepper, salt, and thyme, and whisk well. Pour this mixture in the bowl to make a layer. Bake the quiche pans in a preheated oven at 350 degrees for 25 minutes until it becomes puffy. Examine it with the knife test. Serve in pieces.

Lunch- Chicken Chowder

Yields	:	2- 3
Preparation time	:	4 hours
Total time	:	4 hours 30 min

Ingredients:

| Chicken thighs | 1 pound |
| Cream cheese | 8 ounce |

Chicken broth	1 cup
Diced tomatoes	1 can
Diced onion	1 small
Diced jalapeno	1
Juiced lime	1
Chopped Cilantro	2 tablespoon
Chopped garlic	1 clove
Liquid smoke	few dashes
Salt	1 teaspoon
Pepper	1 tablespoon
Shredded cheese	for garnishing
Chopped cilantro, lime	for garnishing

Directions:

Collect skinless boneless chicken thighs, cream cheese chicken broth, diced tomatoes, diced onion, diced jalapeno, limejuice, chopped cilantro, garlic clove, chopped, liquid smoke, salt, and pepper. Gather cheddar cheese, chopped cilantro, and lime wedge to garnish. Combine the ingredients of chicken chowder in a Crockpot, set it on high and cook for 4 hours. Open the lid and shred the chicken using forks. Take it out in a plate and garnish using shredded cheese, cilantro, and lime wedge. Serve.

Dinner- Yellow Squash Casserole

Yields	:	2- 3
Preparation time	:	30 min
Total time	:	40 min

Ingredients:

Mayonnaise	2 tablespoon
Eggs	2
Cheddar cheese	1.5 cups
Garlic powder	1 tablespoon
Onions, French fried	4 tablespoon
Yellow squash slices	4 cups

Directions:

Combine mayo, eggs, cheddar cheese, garlic powder, and onions in a bowl. Pour yellow squash slices to coat the pieces. Transfer them onto a baking dish and top them with onions and cheese. Bake it in a preheated oven for 30 minutes at 400F on the middle rack.

Day 28

Breakfast- Keto Nib Cereal

Yields   :   2- 3
Preparation time   :   1 hour
Total time   :   1 hour 10 min

Ingredients:

Chia seeds	½ cup
Water	1 cup
Hemp hearts	4 tablespoon
Psyllium powder	1 tablespoon
Vanilla extract	1 tablespoon
Swerve	1 tablespoon
Cacao nibs	1 tablespoon

Directions:

Collect chia seeds, hemp hearts, psyllium powder, coconut oil, vanilla extract, swerve, and cacao nibs. Combine water and chia seeds in a bowl and keep it aside for 5 minutes. Combine all the ingredients in this bowl, apart from cacao nibs. Blend

120

the mixture, and then add the cacao nibs for bigger chunks. Place two large oven papers on the parchment paper. Flatten the dough with your hands and fingers. Cover it with other oven paper. Use a rolling pin to thin the dough. Peel off the oven paper from top. Place the dough on the cookie sheet. Bake on each side for 15- 20 minutes in a preheated oven at 285 degrees. Take out the cookie sheet from the oven, set aside. Slice the cereal into squares of 1 inche. Serve with almond milk.

Lunch- Zoodles with Soup

Yields	:	8-10 cups
Preparation time	:	15 min
Total time	:	20 min

Ingredients:

Coconut oil	1 tablespoon
Chopped onions	½
Jalapeno	1
Green curry paste	1.5 tablespoon

Minced garlic	2 cloves
Chicken bone broth	6 cups
Coconut milk	15 ounce
Sliced Red pepper	1
Chicken breasts	1 pound
Fish sauce	2 tablespoon
Chopped cilantro	½ cup
Spiralized zucchini	2 medium
Lime wedges	1 lime

Directions:

Heat coconut oil in a saucepan and add onions to sauté for 5 minutes. Add curry paste, jalapeno, and garlic. Sauté for a minute, add coconut milk and chicken broth, and whisk well. Let the mixture boil, and lower the heat. Add chicken, fish sauce, and red pepper. Simmer the heat and cook for 5 minutes. Add cilantro. Put some zoodles into the soup bowls, and pour the soup over them. Zoodles will become tender from the heat of soup. Squeeze lemon and serve.

Dinner- Fat Head Spinach Pizza

Yields	:	2- 3
Preparation time	:	20 min
Total time	:	25 min

Ingredients:

Shredded mozzarella	1.5 cup
Cream cheese	2 tablespoon
Almond flour	¾ cup
Egg	1

Directions:

Microwave shredded mozzarella and cream cheese for 1 minute. Stir and microwave for 30 seconds. Now, add egg, almond flour, and microwave for 30 seconds again, and stir. Make a crust with this dough on a parchment paper. Bake it in a preheated oven for 8 minutes at 425F. Pop the bubbles and bake again for 5 minutes. To make Alfredo sauce, melt parmesan cheese in a sauce pan over medium heat. Stir in whipping cream and add pepper and salt. Simmer the heat and let it thicken. Take another pan to cook mushrooms and garlic with butter. Add spinach and wilt them. Now, spread the sauce the pizza base and spread the vegetables mixture. Add canned white chicken and sprinkle mozzarella cheese. Bake again at the same temperature for 10 minutes. Let cool and serve in slices.

Day 29

Breakfast- Porridge with Hemp Hearts

Yields   :   1
Preparation time :   2 min
Total time   :   5 min

Ingredients:

Almond milk	1 cup
Hemp hearts	½ cup
Flax seeds	2 tablespoon
Chia seeds	1 tablespoon
Stevia	5 drops
Vanilla extract	¾ teaspoon
Ground cinnamon	½ teaspoon
Crushed almonds	¼ cup

Topping:

Hemp hearts	1 tablespoon
Brazil nuts	3

Directions:

Collect non- dairy milk, hemp hearts, flax seeds (freshly ground), chia seeds, alcohol free stevia, vanilla extract, ground cinnamon, and crushed almonds. Collect brazil nuts and hemp hearts for topping. Keeping aside the toppings and crushed almonds. Put all ingredients into a saucepan over medium flame and bring it to boil. After the mixture slightly bubbles, stir and cook for 2 minutes. Take the saucepan off the heat, add crushed almonds, and put it in a bowl. Add toppings and serve.

Lunch- Cream of Bacon Chicken Soup

Yields	:	2
Preparation time	:	30 min
Total time	:	40 min

Ingredients:

Bacon	6 slices
Butter	2 tablespoons

Garlic	2 cloves
Sliced Shiitake mushrooms	3.5 ounces
Water/ Cooking wine	1/3 cup
Almond milk	½ cup
Chicken broth	3 cups
Chopped ribs celery	4
Deboned chicken thighs, skinless	4 pieces
Salt	as per taste
Pepper	as per taste
Chopped parsley	2 tablespoons

Directions:

Melt butter in a soup pot and cook bacon in it over low medium heat. When bacon becomes crispy, take it out of the pot and keep it aside. Put a tablespoon of butter in the pot, melt it, and cook garlic in it. Sauté mushrooms in butter, add wine and cook it until it is reduced to half. Add heavy cream, chicken broth, and coconut milk, and cook them. Add pre-cooked chicken pieces and chopped celery. Lower the heat to simmer and let cook for a while. Season with pepper and salt. Garnish with bacon and parsley. Serve.

Dinner- Baked Bacons Cheese Bombs

Yields	:	3-4
Preparation time	:	45 min
Total time	:	55 min

Ingredients:

Mozzarella cheese	8 ounces
Almond flour	4 tablespoon
Melted butter	4 tablespoon
Husk powder	3 tablespoon
Egg	1 large
Salt	¼ teaspoon
Ground pepper `	¼ teaspoon
Garlic powder	1/8 teaspoon
Onion powder	1/8 teaspoon
Bacon	10 slices
Oil	1 cup for frying

Directions:

Microwave some cheese for 60 seconds to slightly melt it. Melt butter in microwave for 15-20 seconds and pour it into egg and cheese in a bowl. Whisk well and put husk powder, spices, and almond flour. Blend well to make dough. Roll it into the shape of rectangle and fill it with solid cheese. Fold it horizontally into half and then vertically into half to make a smaller rectangle. Now, cut 20 small squares from this rectangle. Wrap these squares in bacon slices and secure them with toothpicks. Bake them in a preheated oven at 375 degrees and then fry them for 1-2 minutes. Take them out from the oils on the paper towels and serve.

Day 30

Breakfast- Keto Nuts Cereal

Yields	:	1
Preparation time	:	5 min
Total time	:	5 min

Ingredients:

Cashews	3 grams
Pumpkin seeds, sprouted	18
Brazil nuts	5 grams
Whole hazel nuts	5 grams
Sunflower seeds	1 tablespoon
Walnut	2 grams
Peanut butter	1 tablespoon
Almond butter	1 tablespoon
Cinnamon	1 teaspoon
Brewed coffee	4 ounce
Vanilla extract	1 teaspoon
Greek yogurt	1 ounce
Flax seeds	1 teaspoon

| Hemp seeds | 1 teaspoon |
| Cinnamon powder | 1 teaspoon |

Directions:

Mix all the nuts in a medium bowl, and cover them with yogurt. Now, add almond butter, peanut butter, hemp seeds, vanilla, cinnamon, and flax seeds. Serve with cold coffee.

Lunch- Chili Chicken Soup

Yields	:	2- 3
Preparation time	:	6 hours
Total time	:	6 hours 20 min

Ingredients:

Unsalted butter	2 tablespoon
Onion	1 medium
Green Pepper	1
Chicken thighs, boneless	8
Bacon	8 slices

Thyme	1 tablespoon
Salt	1 teaspoon
Pepper	1 teaspoon
Minced garlic	1 tablespoon
Coconut	1 tablespoon
Lemon juice	3 tablespoon
Chicken stock	1 cup
Unsweetened coconut milk	1 cup
Tomato paste	3 tablespoon

Directions:

Put some butter in the middle of slow cooker. Add green peppers, sliced onions, and distribute them evenly. Spread chicken thighs, and then small chunks of bacon. Add salt, pepper, coconut flour, and garlic. Add lemon juice, coconut milk, chicken stock, and tomato paste. Set the slow cooker on low and cook for 6 hours. When the chicken soup is ready, break the pieces of chicken, and stir the soup. Take out the soup in bowls and top it with sour cream and cheese.

Dinner- Tomato Shakshuka

Yields	:	2- 3
Preparation time	:	40 min
Total time	:	50 min

Ingredients:

Organic yellow onion	1 large
Red Bell pepper	1
Cherry tomatoes	1.5 pound
Olive oil	¼ cup
Cumin seeds	½ tablespoon
Fresh thyme	2 sprigs
Chopped parsley	1 tablespoon
Cayenne	1 pinch
Salt	as per taste
Organic Eggs	4

Directions:

Collect organic yellow onion, bell pepper, cherry tomatoes, olive oil, cumin seeds, fresh thyme, chopped parsley, cayenne, salt, and eggs. Put the cut tomatoes on a greased cookie sheet, sprinkle sea salt, and bake for 30 minutes in a preheated oven at 350F. Take a deep pan, roast cumin seeds, and add chopped onions and olive oil. Sauté on low heat. Put striped bell peppers and herbs. Add caramelized tomatoes, pepper, and salt. Break a few eggs in the pan and spread them. Cook for 10 minutes on low flame. Take off the heat and serve.

CONCLUSION

After reading this book, you must be feeling relieved about starting the ketogenic diet. The major part of beginning a new diet plan is to *think what to eat* every day. This book relieves you from that issue. Just open this book daily, gather the cooking material, and start cooking; no need of thinking this and that.

Just chill with your friends and family while your body is working on itself to shed extra fat. Everybody will be amazed to see you eating so freely and still getting lean. In just a month, you will be enjoying the attention you get. You might get tired of answering people's queries who will want to know the secret behind your health and glow on your face. There is no need to hide anything and just tell them that you are following this amazing diet called Ketogenic diet.

For those who know about it, will be inspired to adopt it immediately, and those who do not know, will immediately Google about it. In any case, you can be the inspirational factor for many people around you. What are you waiting for? Just get up, go to the kitchen and make something delicious!

135

www.ingramcontent.com/pod-product-compliance
Lightning Source LLC
Chambersburg PA
CBHW070141290526
45789CB00002B/578